HABITS FOR BETTER

EYE HEALTH.

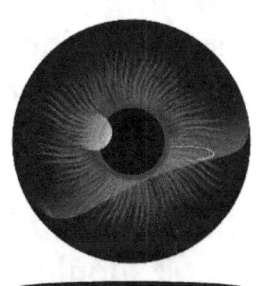

6 MEDICALLY PROVEN STRATEGIES TO BOOST YOUR EYE SIGHT NATURALLY.

TABLE OF CONTENTS

INTRODUCTION

Welcome to "Habits for Improved Eye Health", a complete guide to maintaining optimum eye health via easy but effective lifestyle adjustments.

Our eyes are one of our most treasured and sophisticated organs, allowing us to perceive the world around us in brilliant colors and intricate detail. However, with the popularity of digital gadgets, pollution, and other environmental variables, our eyes are continually subjected to stresses that may lead to visual difficulties and even vision loss.

Fortunately, there are steps we can take to protect and enhance our eye health. In this book, we'll explore routines that may help enhance the health of our eyes, including the right diet, adequate rest, and regular exercise. We'll also dig into ways for lowering eye strain, shield against UV damage, and address common eye disorders.

Whether you're seeking to safeguard your eyesight or conquer eye-related issues, this book provides practical guidance and practical strategies to help you achieve improved eye health. So, let's get started on the path to healthy eyes!

But before we proceed I would like you to meet John, a 32-year-old office worker who has been diagnosed with myopia, also known as nearsightedness.

John's journey with myopia began when he was in high school. He noticed that he had trouble seeing the board during classes and often had to squint to see clearly. At first, he ignored the problem, thinking it was just a passing phase. However, as time went by, his vision continued to deteriorate, and he began experiencing headaches and eye strain.

One day, John decided to visit an optometrist for a comprehensive eye exam. The optometrist confirmed that John had myopia, a common refractive error in which distant objects appear blurry while close-up objects are clear. John was prescribed corrective lenses and was instructed to wear them all the time, including when using a computer or reading a book.

At first, John found it uncomfortable wearing glasses, but he soon realized the benefits they provided. His vision became clearer, and he no longer experienced headaches and eye strain. However, he also realized that he needed to take additional steps to protect his eyes and prevent further deterioration. John made several lifestyle changes to manage his myopia. He started taking regular breaks from his computer screen and using the 20-20-20 rule, which involves looking away from the screen every 20 minutes and focusing on an object 20 feet away for 20 seconds. He also adjusted the lighting in his workspace and ensured that he had adequate ambient light.

Additionally, John started incorporating more eye-healthy foods into his diet, such as leafy greens, citrus fruits, and fish rich in omega-3 fatty acids. He also made a deliberate effort to get adequate sleep, since sleep deprivation may increase myopia symptoms.

Over time, John's myopia has stabilized, and he has not needed to raise the power of his corrective lenses. He continues to practice healthy habits to safeguard his eyes and keep his eyesight.

John's story implies that myopia is a controllable problem with correct diagnosis, treatment, and lifestyle modifications. With the right approach, persons with myopia may have a fulfilling and productive life while maintaining their eyesight for the long term.

PART ONE
WHAT YOU NEED TO KNOW.

WHAT IS SHORT SIGHT SIGHTEDNESS AND LONG SIGHTEDNESS?

Short-sightedness, also known as myopia, is a common vision condition in which distant objects appear blurry, while close-up objects remain clear. It is caused by the shape of the eye, which causes light to focus in front of the retina rather than on it. As a result, distant objects are out of focus, and vision is blurred.

The typical symptoms include;

- Blurred vision while gazing at distant things which shows as difficulty seeing road signs or chalkboards in a classroom
- Squinting to view distant things more clearly.
- Eye strain or tiredness while staring at distant objects over lengthy periods

- Headaches, particularly after reading or using digital gadgets for lengthy periods
- A propensity to sit closer to the TV or hold books closer to the face
- Difficulty seeing well when driving or playing sports
- Trouble seeing at night or in low light settings.

While myopia is typically a benign condition, high levels of myopia can increase the risk of serious eye conditions such as cataracts, glaucoma, and retinal detachment.

It is also crucial to remember that these symptoms may vary in intensity depending on the degree of myopia. If you are experiencing any of these symptoms, then this book is just for you.

long-sightedness, on the other hand, is also known as hyperopia, it is a visual disorder in which far objects will look sharper or more distinct than close-up ones. This is due to an irregularity in the eye's shape, which causes light to concentrate behind the retina rather than on it. As a consequence, close objects appear hazy, and the eyes have to work harder to concentrate on them.

It is often present at birth and may be inherited, however, it can also emerge later in life.

The symptoms of long-sightedness might include eye strain, headaches, and trouble concentrating on close objects. Some individuals may feel blurry vision at all distances, while others may just have a hard time focusing on close-up things.

WHAT YOU SHOULD KNOW ABOUT VISUAL ACUITY.

Visual acuity is a measure of the sharpness and clarity of vision, It is typically the ability of the eye to discern small details and distinguish between different shapes, colors, and patterns at a certain distance.

Visual acuity is expressed as a fraction or ratio, with the numerator representing the distance at which the chart is viewed (usually 20 feet or 6 meters) and the denominator indicating the smallest line of letters that can be read clearly. For example, a person with 20/20 visual acuity can read the smallest line of letters on the chart at a distance of 20 feet, while a person with 20/40 visual acuity can only read letters that are twice as large at the same distance.

Visual acuity can be affected by various factors, such as age, refractive errors (e.g. myopia, hyperopia, or astigmatism), eye diseases, and certain medications.

Maintaining good visual acuity is important for many everyday activities, such as reading, driving, and working. Regular eye exams and early detection of any vision problems can help preserve visual acuity and prevent potential complications.

Achieving and maintaining good visual acuity is the very aim of this book.

PREDISPOSING FACTORS FOR SHORT AND LONG SIGHTEDNESS.

Risk factors for **shortsightedness**, also known as myopia, include:

- Genetics: Family history of myopia is one of the strongest risk factors for developing the condition.

- Age: Myopia usually develops during childhood and tends to stabilize in adulthood, but in some cases, it can continue to progress.

- Prolonged near work: Activities that involve prolonged near work, such as reading or working on a computer, can increase the risk of developing myopia, especially in children.

- Lack of outdoor exposure: medical research have shown that spending more time outdoors and being exposed to natural light can reduce the risk of myopia development and progression.

- Ethnicity: Myopia is more common in certain ethnic groups, such as East Asians.

Risk factors for **long-sightedness**, also known as hyperopia, include:

- Age: Long-sightedness is more common in people over the age of 40.

- Genetics: Family history of hyperopia can increase the risk of developing the condition.

- Medical conditions: Certain medical conditions, such as diabetes or cataracts, can increase the risk of developing hyperopia.

- Eye injuries: Trauma to the eye can cause changes in the shape of the cornea or lens, leading to hyperopia.
- Medications: Certain medications, such as anticholinergics, can cause changes in the way the eye focuses light and increase the risk of hyperopia.

- Eye surgery: Certain kinds of eye surgeries, such as cataract surgery, can increase the risk of developing hyperopia.

Overall, while there are some risk factors beyond our control, there are also many things we can do to lower the chance of developing shortsightedness and long-sightedness as would be explored in part two of this book.

WHAT IS FALSE-SHORT SIGHTEDNESS AND LENS INDUCED MYOPIA.

Pseudomyopia develops when the vision is fixated excessively at close distances. When this occurs, it is difficult to see accurately at a distance, this state is termed false myopia. Pseudomyopia may arise in numerous situations, but it is typical for it to afflict individuals who spend long hours reading or excessively utilizing their near eyesight. fake myopia tends to impact individuals who use a computer or monitor digital displays for several hours to a higher extent.

When a person has pseudomyopia, they not only have problems seeing properly at a distance but also may have additional symptoms in the table:

• Headache.
• Visual fatigue.
• Double vision.
• Dizziness
• Focus issues, while moving their gaze from a distance to a near object.

To accurately separate pseudomyopia from nearsightedness we must take into consideration the following:

• Myopia is a refractive error that occurs when light is projected in front of the retina and not on it. This might arise because the eye is exceptionally long or because the curvature of the cornea and crystalline structure is highly apparent.

• Myopia is caused by the shape of the eye and false myopia is an eye function issue.
While checking the eyes, it might be difficult to discern myopia from fake myopia. This arises because in the eye exam, it is clear whether there is more or less visual strength, but the reason is not established.

• Myopia produces a rise in diopters(unit of measure which denotes the optical power of a lens) throughout the years, but fake myopia may alter in a short period and tends to decrease.

• Even if the symptoms are the same the correction is not the same.

• In real myopia, to acquire excellent vision, we must correct this extra diopter using glasses, contact lenses, or refractive surgery. It is an anatomical issue.

• In the case of fake myopia, what truly exists is a lock-on focus system, and, repairing it in usual ways, simply makes the problems worse. This obstruction generally arises in persons who spend several hours with their eyes focused on near distances.

The best technique to cure fake myopia is via visual therapy. This comprises a series of eye exercises that progressively restore the eye to its natural capacity for accommodation.

DIAGNOSIS OF SHORTSIGHTEDNESS AND LONG SIGHTEDNESS

Shortsightedness and long-sightedness may be diagnosed by a thorough eye examination by an eye care specialist, such as an optometrist or ophthalmologist. During the examination, the eye care physician will do numerous tests to identify the refractive error of the eye.

For shortsightedness, the eye care physician will often use a Snellen chart to determine how well the patient can see items at a distance. If the patient has difficulties seeing items in the distance but can see close-up objects well, they may be diagnosed with myopia.

For long-sightedness, the eye physician may use a near vision chart to determine how well the patient can see items up close. If the patient has difficulties seeing items up close but can see distant objects well, they may be diagnosed with hyperopia.

In addition to these tests, the eye care professional may also employ a retinoscope or autorefractor to assess the refractive error of the eye more precisely. This will assist the eye care specialist establish the right prescription for glasses or contact lenses, if required.

If there are any concerns regarding the health of the eyes or the likelihood of underlying medical disorders, further testing may be requested, such as a dilated eye exam or imaging tests. Overall, a correct diagnosis of shortsightedness or long-sightedness is vital for selecting the proper treatment strategy and sustaining optimal eye health.

ROUTINE CORRECTION FOR THIS EYE DEFECT.

Shortsightedness and long-sightedness may be corrected using numerous procedures, including eyeglasses, contact lenses, and refractive surgery.

For shortsightedness, eyeglasses or contact lenses with a concave (minus) lens are often suggested. These lenses assist to diverge the light entering the eye, which compensates for the elongated shape of the eyeball in myopia. Soft contact lenses or gas-permeable lenses are popular solutions for persons who prefer not to wear glasses.

For long-sightedness, spectacles or contact lenses with a convex (plus) lens are recommended. These lenses serve to concentrate the light entering the eye, which compensates for the shorter shape of the eyeball in hyperopia. Progressive lenses, bifocals, or reading glasses are common solutions for those who require aid with close-up work.

Refractive surgery, like LASIK or PRK, may also be used to rectify shortsightedness and long-sightedness. These surgeries use a laser to reshape the cornea of the eye, which helps to enhance the way the eye focuses light. Unfortunately, not everyone is a suitable candidate for these procedures, and they pose certain risks and possible complications

Overall, the correction of shortsightedness and long-sightedness may considerably enhance eyesight and quality of life. Frequent eye examinations and follow-up visits with an eye care specialist are crucial to guarantee the sustained efficacy of any corrective procedures.

PART TWO
WHAT YOU SHOULD DO.

LIFESTYLE MODIFICATION

Various alterations may be done to improve better eye health and vision for both those with and without eye problems. Some of these alterations include:

For typical individuals:

- Tuning the lighting: Ensure that the lighting is suitable and not too bright or too dark. Avoid direct sunlight and use shades or drapes to prevent glare.

- Taking regular pauses: Taking frequent breaks while working on a computer or reading will help reduce eye strain and weariness. The 20-20-20 rule is advocated, which entails taking a 20-second break every 20 minutes and
- staring at something 20 feet away.

- Keeping a healthy lifestyle: Consuming a balanced diet rich in vitamins and minerals, exercising frequently, and keeping a healthy weight may all contribute to improved eye health.

- Using protective eyewear: Wearing sunglasses or protective glasses during outdoor activities may help protect the eyes from UV radiation, dust, and other particles.

For those with eye defects:

Using corrective lenses: Using eyeglasses or contact lenses may help correct refractive defects such as myopia, hyperopia, or astigmatism, and enhance visual acuity.

Employing assistive technologies: For those with poor vision or a visual impairment, assistive devices such as magnifiers, telescopes, and screen readers may be beneficial in boosting visual function.

Undergoing vision therapy: Vision therapy is a program of exercises and activities aimed to enhance visual function and treat visual disorders such as myopia, hyperopia and also strabismus, amblyopia, or convergence insufficiency.

Considering refractive surgery: For patients with high refractive defects, refractive surgery such as LASIK or PRK might be an option to correct vision and minimize dependency on corrective lenses.

In addition to these improvements, it is crucial to have frequent eye examinations to identify any possible vision impairments or eye disorders early on. Practicing proper eye hygiene and avoiding activities that might strain the eyes, such as smoking or excessive screen time, can also help to improve eye health and vision.

RELEVANCE OF SLEEP TO YOUR EYE.

Sleep has a key part in maintaining excellent overall health, and this includes the health of our eyes. These are some reasons why enough sleep is vital for eye health:

Relieves Eye Strain: Sleep is a natural approach to ease eye strain, especially if you spend a lot of time in front of a computer or other digital devices. While you sleep, your eyes receive a respite from the frequent exposure to blue light, which may induce eye tiredness and strain.

Prevents Dry Eyes: During sleep, the body generates less tears, which may contribute to dry eyes. Nevertheless, getting adequate sleep may help avoid this by enabling the eyes to relax and minimizing the likelihood of having dry eyes.

Reduces the Risk of Eye Diseases: Research has shown that a lack of sleep might raise the risk of certain eye illnesses, such as glaucoma, macular degeneration, and diabetic retinopathy. Sufficient sleep is vital for preserving the health of the retina and avoiding damage to the optic nerve.

Supports Healing: Sleep is a period when the body heals and regenerates itself, including the eyes. Obtaining adequate sleep helps aid recovery of any small injuries or infections that may arise in or around the eyes.

Increases Attention and Concentration: Sufficient sleep is vital for enhancing focus and concentration, which may help minimize eye strain and weariness. This is especially crucial for persons who conduct occupations that need a lot of visual attention, such as driving, reading, or working on a computer.

In short, obtaining adequate sleep is vital for maintaining excellent eye health. It may help reduce eye strain, dry eyes, and eye illnesses, promote healing, and increase focus and attention. If you have difficulties sleeping, speak to your healthcare professional about ways for changing your sleep

patterns.

EYE SUPPLEMENTS WITH NATURAL INGREDIENTS.

There are several eye supplements available on the market that include natural substances, which are considered to enhance eye health and improve visual performance. These are some popular natural components found in eye supplements and their potential benefits:

Lutein and Zeaxanthin: These are carotenoids that are present in high quantities in the macula of the eye. They serve as antioxidants, protecting the eyes from damage caused by free radicals and UV radiation. They are also thought to aid enhance visual acuity, contrast sensitivity, and lessen the risk of age-related macular degeneration (AMD).

Omega-3 Fatty Acids: They are necessary fatty acids that are crucial for supporting the integrity of cell membranes in the eye. They also contain anti-inflammatory effects, which may help minimize the risk of eye illnesses such as dry eye syndrome and AMD.

Vitamin C: This antioxidant vitamin is crucial for preserving the integrity of the eye's blood vessels and avoiding oxidative damage to the eye. It is also thought to lessen the risk of cataracts.

Vitamin E: This fat-soluble vitamin has antioxidant qualities and is crucial for protecting the cells of the eye from damage caused by free radicals. It is also thought to lessen the risk of cataracts and AMD.

Zinc: This mineral is crucial for maintaining the health of the retina and is involved in the synthesis of melanin, a pigment that shields the eye from UV rays. It is also thought to lessen the risk of AMD.

Bilberry: This is a fruit that is high in anthocyanins, which are antioxidants that may help protect the eyes from oxidative damage and lessen the incidence of AMD.

It is crucial to remember that although natural chemicals included in eye supplements might be good for eye health, they should not substitute a balanced diet and lifestyle. It is always suggested to contact with a healthcare practitioner before beginning any new supplement regimen, particularly if you have any underlying medical concerns or are taking medication.

ROLES OF NUTRITIONALLY DENSE MEALS.

1. Several fish are good providers of omega-3 fatty acids.

Oily fish are fish that contain oil in their gut and body tissue, therefore eating them delivers greater doses of omega-3-rich fish oil. The fish that provides the greatest beneficial quantities of omega-3s include

- tuna
- salmon
- trout
- mackerel
- sardines
- anchovies
- herring

Several studies have suggested that fish oil helps reverse dry eye, especially dry eye induced by spending too much time on a computer.

2. Nuts and legumes

Nuts are also high in omega-3 fatty acids. Nuts also have a high quantity of vitamin E, which helps protect the eye from age-related damage.

Nuts are available for purchase in most grocery shops and online. Nuts and legumes that are excellent for eye health include:

- walnuts
- Brazil nuts
- cashews
- peanuts
- lentils

3. Like nuts and legumes, seeds are high in omega-3s and are a great source of vitamin E.

Seeds are available for purchase at most grocery shops and online. Seeds rich in omega-3 include:

chia seeds

flax seeds

hemp seeds

4. Citrus fruits

Citrus fruits are high in vitamin C. Much like vitamin E, vitamin C is an antioxidant that is suggested by the AOA to counteract age-related eye damage.

Vitamin C-rich citrus fruits include:

lemons

oranges

grapefruits

5. Leafy green veggies

Leafy green vegetables are high in both lutein and zeaxanthin and are also a strong source of eye-friendly vitamin C.

Well-known leafy greens include:

spinach

skale

collards

6. Carrots

Carrots are rich in both Vitamin A and beta carotene. Beta carotene gives carrots their orange hue.

Vitamin A plays a crucial part in eyesight. It is a component of protein called rhodopsin, which allows the retina to absorb light.

7. Sweet potatoes

Like carrots, sweet potatoes are high in beta carotene. They are also a strong source of the antioxidant vitamin E.

8. Beef

Beef is rich in zinc, which can improve long-term eye health. Zinc may help postpone age-related visual loss and macular degeneration.

The eye itself has large quantities of zinc, notably in the retina, and the vascular tissue surrounding the retina.

Meats such as chicken breast and pig loin also contain zinc,

9. Eggs

Eggs are a rich source of lutein and zeaxanthin, which may lessen the risk of age-related visual loss. Eggs are also rich providers of vitamins C and E, and zinc.

10. Water, yes water may come as no surprise as fluid necessary to existence is also critical to eye health.

Drinking plenty of water can prevent dehydration, which may reduce the symptoms of dry eyes.

EXERCISES RELEVANT FOR EYE HEALTH

Eye exercises may be effective for maintaining excellent eye health and minimizing eye strain caused by continuous use of digital gadgets or other activities that demand high visual attention. Here are some exercises that may be helpful:

Blinking: Blinking frequently might help keep the eyes moisturized and decrease dryness and discomfort. Try blinking every 4-5 seconds for a minute or two to help relax the eyes.

Focusing: Concentrate on a thing at a distance, then move your attention to an object up close. Perform this exercise multiple times to help strengthen the eye muscles.

Palming: Rub your hands together to warm them up, then lay them over your eyes for a few minutes to assist relax the eyes and minimize eye strain.

Figure 8s: Imagine a giant figure 8 in front of you, then trace it with your eyes. This practice may assist improve eye coordination and strengthen eye muscles.

Eye rotations: Glance up, then down, then left, then right, then move your eyes in a circular motion. Repeat multiple rounds to help develop eye muscle flexibility.

Near-to-far focusing: Keep an item up close, then progressively move it farther away while retaining your attention on it. Perform this exercise multiple times to help increase attention and minimize eye strain.

STRESS REDUCTION STRATEGY

Stress is a major source of eye strain, which may lead to a variety of eye disorders including dry eyes, headaches, and impaired vision. These are some stress reduction practices that may assist enhance eye health:

Mindfulness meditation: Mindfulness meditation entails concentrating on the present moment without judgment. Frequent practice of mindfulness meditation has been demonstrated to decrease stress and anxiety, which may assist minimize eye strain.

Yoga: Doing yoga may help relieve stress and tension in the body, particularly the eyes. Certain eye movements within yoga, such as cyc rotations and palming, may also aid enhance eye health.

Exercise: Regular exercise may help decrease stress and enhance general health, which can benefit the eyes. Exercise also helps to boost blood flow and oxygen to the eyes, which may help minimize eye strain and weariness.

Relaxation approaches: Relaxation techniques such as deep breathing, progressive muscle relaxation, and visualization may help decrease stress and tension in the body, which can improve the eyes.

Digital detox: Taking pauses from digital devices such as computers, cellphones, and tablets might help minimize eye strain and weariness. It is advisable to take a break every 20 minutes and look away from the computer to avoid eye strain.

Time in nature: Spending time in nature has been demonstrated to relieve stress and promote mental and physical health. This may help minimize eye strain and enhance overall eye health.

JUDICIOUS USE OF PRESCRIPTION LENSES.

Prescription lenses are a common way to correct refractive errors such as myopia (nearsightedness), hyperopia (farsightedness), and astigmatism. While prescription lenses can improve vision and quality of life, it is important to use them judiciously to avoid potential risks and complications. Here are some important considerations for the judicious use of prescription lenses:

Proper fitting: Proper fitting of prescription lenses is essential to ensure optimal vision correction and comfort. An improperly fitted lens can cause discomfort, eye strain, headaches, and even damage to the eyes.

Regular eye exams: It is important to have regular eye exams to ensure that your prescription is up-to-date and to detect any changes in your eye health. Your eye doctor can also advise you on the appropriate use of prescription lenses.

Proper care: Proper care of prescription lenses is important to maintain their effectiveness and to reduce the risk of infection or other complications. This includes cleaning the lenses regularly, storing them properly, and replacing them as recommended by your eye doctor.

Limiting use: Overuse of prescription lenses, especially for activities such as reading or using digital devices for extended periods of time, can lead to eye strain, headaches, and other problems. It is important to take breaks and practice good eye habits such as blinking regularly and maintaining proper posture.

Avoiding overcorrection: Overcorrection with prescription lenses can lead to further eye strain and discomfort. It is important to follow your eye doctor's recommendations for the appropriate level of correction

Considering alternative options: In some cases, alternative options such as orthokeratology (corneal reshaping), vision therapy, or refractive surgery may be appropriate for certain individuals. It is crucial to examine these alternatives with your eye doctor to identify the best course of action for your unique circumstances.

THE END.

www.ingramcontent.com/pod-product-compliance
Lightning Source LLC
Chambersburg PA
CBHW071146220526
45467CB00015B/1989